Terms and Conditions

LEGAL NOTICE

Table Of Contents

Foreword

Do you love a drink from time to time? A lot of us do, often when socializing with acquaintances and loved ones. Drinking may be beneficial or harmful, depending upon your age and health status, and, naturally, how much you drink.

Alcohol addiction is something that can't be formed in simple terms. Alcohol addiction in general refers to the condition that is an obsession to continue drinking even if it harms health. Alcoholism means you don't have any control over intake despite being well aware of the damaging consequences.

An alcoholic individual drinks even if he happens to get into alcohol related troubles like drunk driving, losing his job, etcetera.

Not everyone who takes in alcohol is an alcoholic. An individual who takes in alcohol in controlled quantities and is able to say no when he doesn't want to drink isn't termed alcohol-dependent. He or she is simply a social drinker.

For anybody who drinks, this book offers valuable, research-based info. What do you think of taking a look at your drinking habits and how they might affect your health? This can help you get started.

Alcohol-No-More

Finally Free Yourself From Alcoholic Waste And Live A Healthy Life

Chapter 1:

The Basics On Alcohol Use

Synopsis

Do you realize that national surveys have suggested that nearly fourteen-million Americans, that's one in thirteen grownups, abuse alcohol or are alcoholic? For many adults, moderate alcohol use (1-2 drinks daily for men and 1 drink daily for women and elderly) isn't harmful.

As a matter of fact, moderate alcohol use has indicated to have a favorable effect on cardiac health, and may be a pleasant plus to social affairs. But, unhealthy alcohol abuse may be life-threatening.

Heavy drinking has been evidenced to step-up one's risk for particular cancers, especially liver, esophagus, throat, and larynx.

Additionally, heavy drinking may induce cirrhosis of the liver, brain damage, and damage to the immune system. Drinking step-ups one's risk of death from a car crash or recreational/occupational injury, and may induce severe economic hardship if one's drinking conduct affects one's power to maintain a steady job.

Facts You Need To Look At

Alcoholism is a serious, often under-recognized, national disease. UR students should learn to recognize the signs and symptoms of alcoholism, and that affected individuals are given appropriate support and assistance before it is too late.
Alcohol Use

Alcohol Abuse

According to the NIAAA, alcohol abuse is outlined as a pattern of drinking that results in one or more of the accompanying situations inside a 12-month time period:

- Failure to accomplish major work, school, or household responsibilities
- Drinking in spots that are physically unsafe, like while driving a car or controlling machinery
- Having repeating alcohol-related legal troubles, like being arrested for driving under the influence of alcohol or for physically wounding somebody while drunk
- Continued drinking in spite of having ongoing relationship troubles that are caused or aggravated by the drinking

When an individual abuses alcohol s/he utilizes it with the sole purpose of getting intoxicated, utilizes it in such a way that it leads to a formula of damaging consequences, and/or experiences harm directly related to and induced by his/her usage of alcohol. A few examples of alcohol-related harms generally experienced by people who abuse alcohol are: blacking out, vomiting, getting into a scrap, and/or memory lapse. Such people will have a BAC higher than 0.06.

Alcohol Dependence

When a person gets physically dependent upon a substance s/he experiences cravings and an irresistible impulse to utilize it. If s/he doesn't utilize the substance, s/he will go through withdrawal. Individuals who are dependent upon alcohol are obsessed with the utilization of the substance, and its utilization becomes a daily/weekly precedence.

Pupils who are alcohol dependent frequently schedule solely late classes, lose the power to predict how much they're going to drink in a evening (lack of self-command), experience lots of blackouts, sneak drinks in order to conceal how much they really consume from close acquaintances and loved ones, drink before going out , and acquire/maintain a high tolerance.

Additionally, any efforts utilized to cut back drinking are unsuccessful. While a lot of dependent pupils feel as if his/her drinking troubles will cease with graduation from college, these people are frequently sadly mistaken. Dependence is a serious medical issue that requires time, diligence, and support to defeat. But, help is available.

Alcoholism

Alcoholism is the disease that happens when a person gets physically dependent on/addicted to alcohol. Frequently non-alcoholics don't comprehend why an alcoholic can't overrule their desire to drink with

self-control or dedication. Regrettably, it isn't that easy. Alcoholics hunger alcohol just as humans crave food or water, and will literally feel an obsession to drink in order to endure.

Alcoholics lose the power to limit their intake of alcohol, as well as to confine their drinking to particular occasions and/or celebrations. Without alcohol, alcoholics experience a period of withdrawal, like that of person addicted to "hard drug" like cocaine or heroin, with symptoms like nausea, sweating, shakiness, tension, and insomnia.

Over time one's tolerance will expand, causing an alcoholic to consume a greater and greater amount of alcohol in order to pacify their physical cravings and get the "high".

Research demonstrates that the risk of acquiring alcoholism tends to run in families. While genes surely play a role, lifestyle is truly the determinant. Alcoholism may generally be avoided with safe, continual supervising of alcohol intake.

Discerning An Issue

Discerning an issue is unique to every individual drinker. Different individuals might feel the negative effects of alcohol misuse/abuse after consuming different quantities of alcohol over variable lengths of time, and no 2 drinkers are precisely alike.

In the first place, concerned persons ought to ask themselves the accompanying questions.

- Do you drink since you have troubles? To unwind?
- Do you drink if you get angry at others, your friends or family?

- Do you want to drink alone, instead of with other people?
- Are your grades beginning to drop off? Are you goldbricking on your job?
- Did you ever try to stop drinking or drink less - and fail?
- Have you started to drink in the morning, prior to school or work?
- Do you swig your drinks?
- Do you ever lose memories ascribable to your drinking?
- Do you fake your drinking?
- Do you get into trouble when you are drinking?
- Do you become drunk when you drink, even if you don't intend to?

If you discover that you've answered yes to one or more of the above questions you might either have or be developing an alcohol-related issue.

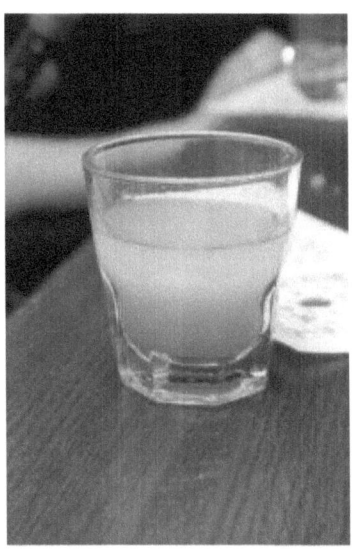

Chapter 2:

Are You Ready To Quit

Synopsis

Are you prepared to alter your drinking?

How many times have you stated to yourself "I can't take this any longer, I need to stop drinking alcohol"? If you're addicted to alcohol you've likely said this to yourself and possibly other people more times than you are able to count. The query is – are you truly ready to stop?

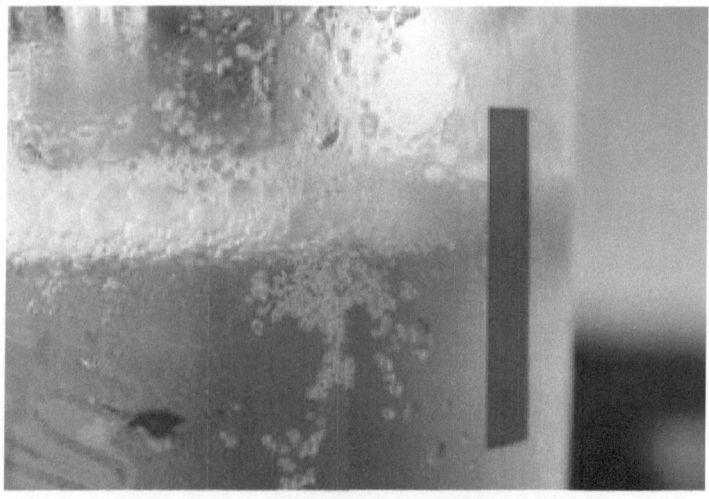

Understand What Stage You Are At And What To Do

The reality of the issue and your initial obstacle to putting that booze down is the addicted part of you, isn't going to join forces with the part that wants to stop. The dependant part of you will never desire to quit drinking.

The healthy part of you realizes the damage you're causing from alcohol and recognizes this state of affairs has gone way over the line, but once more, the dependant part of you will never wish to stop permanently.

Life without alcohol is too dreadful a consideration if you are able to even picture it at all. And walking off from something that has become such an inherent piece of your life with predictable (consequently consoling on some level) results is a fearful step into the strange.

First of all you have to take stock of your state of affairs. You have to be really honest with yourself and take a full close up look at the harm alcohol has induced in your life. And understand that if you carry on drinking, your life will carry on to go downhill.

For a few of the more operational drinkers, your life might look great from the outside. But those who are apparently "pulling it off" are the ones who are more likely to finally run into severe health troubles or even death from the common drinking illnesses like cirrhosis, merely because they don't feel the urging to quit drinking as soon as the drinker who's "knocked down" by alcohol earlier in their drinking .

This brand of drinker is bearing a multitude of effects much sooner than the functional drinker and becoming more desperate and driven as a result is more probable to look for help sooner.

If drinking is taking a severe toll on you and after you've decided you've had enough of the ongoing issues alcohol addiction is inducing for you, you'll need not only the bravery to make your start, but likewise to choose a great strategy in the form of help to free yourself from the steady, ceaseless drinking that will unavoidably take away everything you care about from your lifetime.

If you're considering altering your drinking, you'll have to decide whether to cut back or to stop.

It's a great idea to talk over different alternatives with a physician, an acquaintance, or somebody else you trust.

Stopping is strongly suggested if you:

- Attempt cutting back but can't stay inside the limits you set
- Have experienced an alcohol use disorder or now have symptoms
- Have a physical or mental circumstance that is caused or aggravated by drinking
- Are taking a medicine that interacts with alcohol
- Are or might become pregnant

If none of the circumstances above apply to you, then talk with your physician to ascertain whether you ought to cut back or quit based on factors like:

- Family history of alcohol issues
- Your age
- Whether you've had drinking-related wounds
- Symptoms like sleep disorders and sexual dysfunction

If you choose whether to cut down or stop and make a change plan. Don't be amazed if you carry on to have mixed feelings. You might need to redo your decision many times before becoming comfortable with it.

Even when you have devoted yourself to making an alteration, you still might have mixed feelings at times. Making a written "change plan" will help you to set your goals, why you desire to reach them, and how you plan to do it.

A sample form is provided here.

Goal: (select one)

_____I want to drink no more   drink(s) on any day and no than _____   more than_____drink(s) per week.

_____I want to stop drinking.

Timing:

I will start on this date: _____

Reasons:

My most important reasons to make these changes are:

_____

    _____

    _____

Strategy

I will use these strategies:

    _____

    _____

    _____

People:

The people who can assist me are (names and how they can help):

    _____

    _____

    _____

    _____

Signs of success:

I will know my plan is working if:

    _____

    _____

Possible roadblocks:

Some things that might interfere—and how I'll handle them:

Roadblocks

    _____

_____

How I'll handle them

_____

_____

If you feel you are not yet ready to take any action, consider these suggestions in the meantime:

- Keep track of how frequently and how much you're drinking
- Observe how drinking affects you
- Make or refashion a list of pros and cons about modifying behavior
- Deal with additional priorities that might be in the way
- Ask for support from your physician, a acquaintance, or somebody else you trust
- Consider steps to be safe.

Keep Track

Date	Situation (what's going on)	Sort	Amount	Consequences

Chapter 3:

If You Start With Cutting Back

Synopsis

Little changes may make a huge difference in cutting back your chances of having alcohol-related issues. Whatsoever techniques you pick out, give them an impartial trial. If one plan of attack doesn't work, attempt something else. But if you have not made advancement in cutting back after 2 to 3 calendar months, you may need to stop drinking altogether, look for professional help, or both.

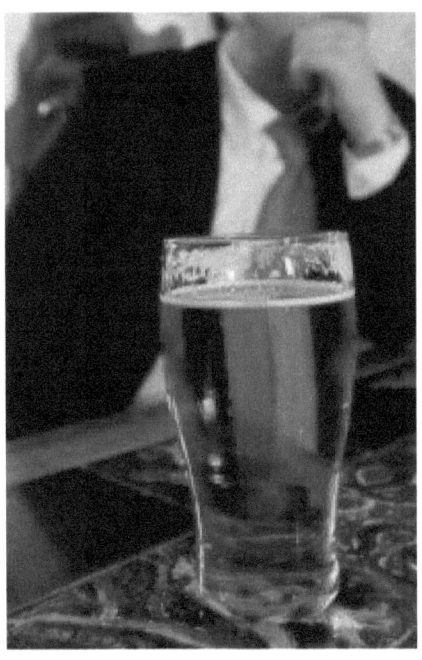

Beginning Tips

Here are a few techniques to try out, and you'll be able to add your own at the end. Mark off maybe 2 or 3 to attempt in the following week or two.

Keep a record.

Keep a record of how much you are drinking. Discover a way that works for you, carry around drinking tracker cards in your wallet (in the previous chapter), make checks on a kitchen calendar, or record notations in a mobile phone notepad or PDA. Making note of every drink prior to you drinking it might help you slow down when you need to.

Tally and measure.

Understand the standard drink sizes so you are able to tally your drinks precisely. Measure drinks at home. Away from home, it may be hard to keep track, particularly with mixed drinks, and from time to time, you might be getting more alcohol than you believe. With wine, you might need to ask the host or server not to "top off" a partly filled glass.

Many people are amazed to learn what counts as a drink. In the U.S., a "standard" drink is any drink that bears about 0.6 fluid ounces or 14 grams of "pure" alcohol. Although the drinks here are different sizes,

each contains about the same amount of alcohol and counts as a single standard drink.

12 fl oz of regular beer =

8-9 fl oz of malt liquor =

5 fl oz of table wine =

3-4 oz of fortified wine =

2-3 oz of cordial, liqueur, or aperitif =

1.5 oz of brandy (a single jigger or shot) =

1.5 fl oz shot of 80-proof spirits ("hard liquor")

Arrange goals.

Select how many days a week you wish to drink and how many drinks you'll consume on those days. It's a great idea to have a few days when you do not drink. Drinkers with the lowest rates of alcohol use disorders remain within the low-risk limits.

- "Low risk" isn't "no risk." Even inside these limits, drinkers may have issues if they drink too quickly, have ill health, or are older (both men and women over sixty-five are commonly advised to have no more than 3 drinks on any day and 7 per week). Based on your wellness and how alcohol affects you, you might need to drink less or not at all.

Pace and distance.

If you do drink, pace yourself. Sip bit-by-bit. Have no more than one standard drink with alcohol per hour. Use "drink spacers"—make every other drink a non-alcoholic one, like water, soda, or juice.

Put in food.

Don't drink on an empty-bellied stomach. Consume some food so the alcohol will be soaked up into your system more slowly.

Discover alternatives.

If drinking has used up a lot of your time, then fill spare time by developing fresh, healthy activities, hobbies, and relationships, or regenerating ones you've missed. If you've counted on alcohol to be more comfortable in sociable situations, handle moods, or cope with issues, then seek other, good for you ways to deal with those areas of your life.

Prevent "triggers."

What triggers your impulse to drink? If particular individuals or places make you drink even when you don't wish to, attempt to avoid them. If particular activities, times of day, or feelings touch off the urge, plan something else to do rather than drinking. If drinking at home is an issue, keep little or no alcohol there.

Plan to manage urges.

When you can't avoid a trigger and an impulse hits, think about these options: Remind yourself of your causes for changing (it may help to carry them in writing or store them in an electronic message you are able to access easily).

Or talk things over with somebody you trust. Or get involved with a fit, distracting activity, like physical exercise or a hobby that doesn't call for drinking. Or, rather than fighting the feeling, accept it and ride it out without buckling under, knowing that it will shortly crest like a wave and pass.

Also, see the following chapters to help you handle urges to drink.

Understand your "no."

You're likely to be offered up a drink at times when you don't need one. Have a civil, convincing "no, thanks" prepared. The quicker you are able to say no to these offers, the less likely you are to buckle under. If you waver, it allows you time to consider excuses to go along. Also, see the following chapters to help you build up drink refusal skills.

List your own strategies:

_____

_____

Chapter 4:

Handling Urges

Synopsis

The accompanying tips offer suggestions to support you in your determination to cut back or stop drinking. They may be used with counseling or therapy and are not meant as a replacement for professional help. If you decide to try them on your own and at any point feel you require more help, then seek support.

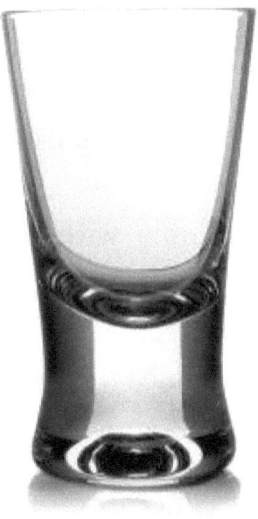

Give Yourself A Little Help

Managing urges to drink

As you alter your drinking, it's common place and standard to have urges or a hungering for alcohol. The words "urge" and "craving" refer to a blanket range of ideas, physical sensations, or emotions that entice you to drink, even though you've at least a little desire not to. You might feel an uncomfortable pulled in 2 directions or sense a loss of command.

As luck would have it, urges to drink are transitory, predictable, and controllable. Here we offer a recognize-avoid-cope plan of attack generally utilized in cognitive behavioral therapy, which helps individuals alter unhelpful thinking patterns and responses.

With time, and by using fresh reactions, you'll discover that your urges to drink will lose power, and you'll acquire confidence in your power to deal with urges that might still arise from time to time.

If you're having a really difficult time with urges, or don't make progress with the techniques here after a couple of weeks, then consult a physician or therapist for support. Additionally, some new, non-habit forming medicines may reduce the desire to drink or lessen the reinforcing effect of drinking so it's simpler to stop.

Acknowledge 2 sorts of "triggers"

An impulse to drink may be set off by outside triggers in the surroundings and internal ones inside yourself.

- Outside triggers are individuals, places, things, or times of day that provide drinking opportunities or prompt you about drinking. These "risky situations" are more conspicuous, predictable, and avoidable than inner triggers.

- Inner triggers may be puzzling as the urge to drink simply appears to "pop up." But if you hesitate to consider it when it occurs, you'll discover that the urge might have been set off by a passing thought, a positive emotion like excitement, a negative emotion like frustration, or a physical sensation like a headache, tension, or nervousness.

Think about tracking and examining your urges to drink for a few weeks. This will help you get more aware of when and how you go through urges, what sparks them, and ways to prevent or control them.

Prevent risky situations

In a lot of cases, your best technique will be to prevent taking the chance that you'll have an impulse, then slip and drink. At home, hold little or no alcohol. Socially, prevent activities demanding drinking. If you feel shamefaced about turning down an invitation, prompt yourself that you're not necessarily saying "forever."

If the urges subside or become more manageable, you might decide to ease bit by bit into a few situations you now decide to avoid. Meanwhile, you are able to stay connected with friends by proposing alternative activities that don't call for drinking.

Contend with triggers you can't prevent

It's not possible to avoid all risky situations or to block inner triggers, so you'll require a range of techniques to address impulses to drink.

Here are a few options:

- Prompt yourself of your grounds for making a change. Carry around your top reasons on a wallet card or in an electronic message that you are able to access easily, like a cell phone notepad entry or a saved e-mail.

- Talk it through with somebody you trust. Have a trusted acquaintance on standby for a telephone call, or bring one along to risky situations.

- Distract yourself with a fit, alternate activity. For different states of affairs, come up with engaging short, mid-range, and longer choices, like texting or calling somebody, watching short net video, lifting weights to audio, showering, meditating, taking a walk, or doing a spare-time activity.

- Take exception to the thought that drives the impulse. Stop it, study the fault in it, and substitute it. Illustration: "It couldn't hurt to have one tiny drink. Hold off a minute—what am I thinking? One may hurt, as I've seen 'simply one' lead to lots more. I'm sticking to my selection not to drink."

- Ride it out without buckling under. Rather than fighting an impulse, accept it as common place and temporary. As you ride it out, bear in mind that it will soon peak like an ocean wave and blow over.

- Leave risky situations rapidly and graciously. It helps to plan your escape beforehand.

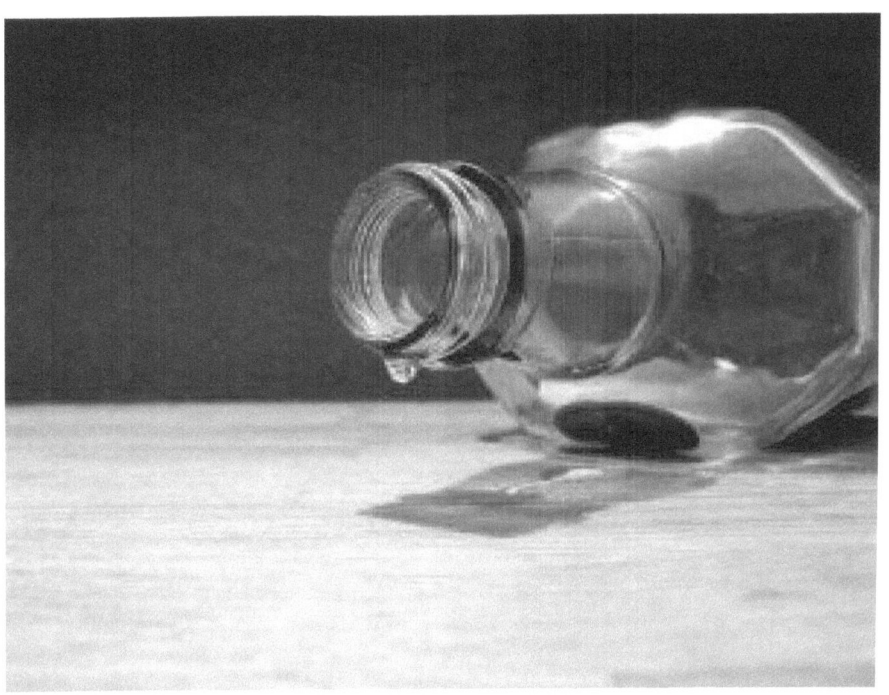

Chapter 5:

Saying No Skills

Synopsis

Even if you're devoted to altering your drinking, "social pressure" to drink from acquaintances or other people may make it difficult to cut down or stop. This chapter provides a recognize-avoid-cope plan of attack commonly utilized in cognitive-behavioral therapy, which helps individuals alter unhelpful thinking patterns and responses.

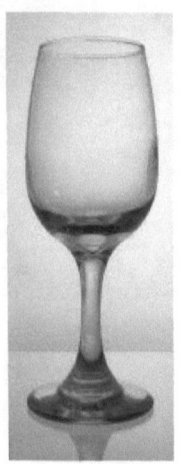

Contend with situations you can't avoid (also worth repeating)

Recognize your "no"

If you realize alcohol will be served, it's crucial to have a few resistance techniques lined up beforehand. If you anticipate to be offered a drink, you'll have to be ready to give up a convincing "no thanks." Your goal is to be clear-cut and steadfast, yet friendly and respectful. Prevent long explanations and faint excuses, as they tend to extend the discussion and supply more of an opportunity to buckle under.

Here are a few other points to bear in mind:

- Don't waver, as that will give you the opportunity to dream up reasons to go along
- Look directly at the individual and attain eye contact
- Keep your reaction short, clear up, and simple

The individual offering you a drink might not know you're attempting to cut back or quit, and his or her level of insistency might vary. It's a great idea to plan a series of reactions in case the individual persists, from an easy refusal to a more self-assertive reply.

Think about a sequence like this:

- No, thanks.
- No, thank you, I don't wish to.

- You know, I'm (cutting down/not drinking) now (to get fitter/to take care of myself/as my physician said to). I'd truly appreciate it if you would help me out.

You are able to also try the "broken record" technique. Every time the individual makes a statement, you are able to simply repeat the same short, clean-cut response. You may wish to acknowledge some part of the individuals points ("I hear you...") and then return to your broken-record reply ("...but no thank you"). And if words flunk, you are able to walk away.

Script and rehearse your "no"

A lot of individuals are amazed at how hard it may be to say no the first couple of times. You may establish confidence by scripting and rehearsing your lines. First of all imagine the situation and the individual who's putting up the drink. Then write both what the individual will say and how you'll answer, whether it's a broken record technique (mentioned above) or your own unique plan of attack.

Repeat it out loud to get comfortable with your choice of words and delivery. Likewise, think about asking a supportive individual to role-play with you, somebody who would offer truthful pressure to drink and truthful feedback about your answers. Whether you rehearse through fabricated or real life experiences, you'll learn as you go. Keep at it, and your tools will grow over time.

Attempt additional techniques

In addition to being fixed with your "no thank you," think about these techniques:

- Have non-alcoholic drinks constantly in hand if you're stopping, or as "drink spacers" between drinks if you're cutting down
- Keep a record of each drink if you're cutting down so you remain inside your limits
- Invite support from other people to contend with temptation
- Plan an escape if the enticement gets too big
- Ask other people to refrain from pressuring you or drinking in your presence (this may be difficult)

If you've successfully declined drink offers before, then remember what worked and build on it.

Remember, it's your option

How you consider any decision to alter your habits may impact your success. A lot of individuals who choose to cut down or stop drinking think, "I'm not allowed to drink," as if an outside authority were enforcing rules. Thoughts like this may breed bitterness and make it easier to buckle under. It's crucial to challenge this sort of thinking by telling yourself that you're in charge, that you know how you wish your life to be, and that you've chosen to make a change.

Likewise, you might worry about how other people will respond or view you if you make a shift. Once again, challenge these thoughts by recalling that it's your life and your option, and that your determination ought to be respected.

Chapter 6:

Treatment To Deal With Alcohol Abuse

Synopsis

Whether you decide to go to rehab, rely on self-help programs, get therapy, or take a self-reliant treatment plan of attack, support is crucial. Don't attempt to go it alone. Recovering from alcoholism is much simpler when you have individuals you are able to lean on for encouragement, comfort, and counsel.

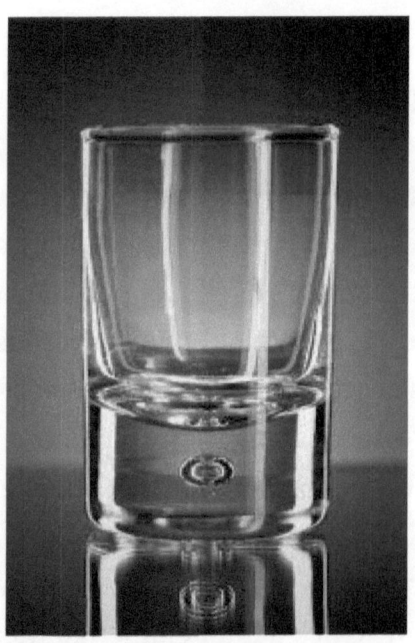

A Few Options

Support may come from loved ones, acquaintances, counselors, other recovering alcoholics, your health professional, and individuals from your faith community.

Lean against close acquaintances and loved ones – Having the support of acquaintances and loved ones is a priceless asset in recovery. If you're reluctant to turn to your family because you've let them down earlier, think about going to counseling or therapy.

Construct a sober societal network – If your former social life centered on alcohol, you might need to make a few fresh connections. It's crucial to have sober acquaintances that will support your recovery. Attempt taking a class, joining a church or a civic group, volunteering, or going to events in your community.

Think about moving in to a sober living home. Sober living homes supply a safe, supportive place to live while you're recovering from alcohol. They are a great choice if you don't have a stable household or an alcohol -free living environment to go to.

Make meetings a precedence – link up with a recovery support group and attend meetings on a regular basis. Spending time with individuals who comprehend precisely what you're going through may be very healing. You are able to likewise benefit from the shared experiences of the group members and learn what other people have done to stay sober.

Alcoholics Anonymous (AA) is the most long-familiar and widely available self-help group for alcoholics in treatment and recovery.

A key component of a 12-step program is picking a sponsor. A sponsor is a former user who has time and experience staying sober and may provide support when you're dealing with the impulse to use.

Research treatment choices

If you choose that you'd like to see a mental health care provider and capitalize on the latest dependency therapies, it's time to research your treatment choices. As you think about the options, bear the following in mind:

- There's no magical bullet or individual treatment that works for everybody. When thinking about a program, remember that everyone's needs are assorted. Alcohol addiction treatment ought to be custom-made to your unique issues and situation. It's crucial that you find a program that feels correct.
- Treatment ought to address more than simply your alcohol abuse. Addiction affects your entire life, including your kinships, job, health, and psychological welfare.
- Treatment success depends upon examining the way alcohol abuse has affected you and developing a fresh way of living.

Dedication and follow-through are chief. Recovering from alcoholism isn't a quick and simple process. As a whole, the longer and more intense the alcohol utilization, the longer and more intense the treatment you'll require. However regardless of the treatment program's length in weeks or months, long-run follow through care is imperative to recovery.

There are a lot of places to turn for help. Not everyone requires medically managed detox or an extended stretch in rehab. The level of care you require depends upon your age, alcohol use history, and additional medical or psychiatric circumstances. In addition to physicians and psychologists, a lot of clergy members, caseworkers, and counselors provide addiction treatment services.

While evaluating the a lot of types of alcohol treatment programs, recall that everyone's needs are different. A quality treatment plan not only addresses the alcohol abuse, it likewise addresses the emotional pain and additional life issues that contribute to your addiction.

As you look for help for alcohol addiction, it's likewise crucial to get treatment for any additional medical or psychological issues you're going through.

Alcohol abuse oftentimes goes hand in hand with other mental health issues, including anxiety, depression, ADD, and manic depression. In a lot cases, the drinking is an attempt to self-medicate. When these issues coincide, recovery depends upon treating them both.

Chapter 7:

Alternative Ways To Deal With Alcohol Abuse

Synopsis

Alternative treatment for alcoholism has advanced in fame in recent times. This treatment strategy involves blending in both traditional and modern scientific strategies of treatment for certain symptoms. Different than treatment of other diseases alcoholism ought to be treated with extra care. Effort must be taken to produce surroundings which are free of tension.

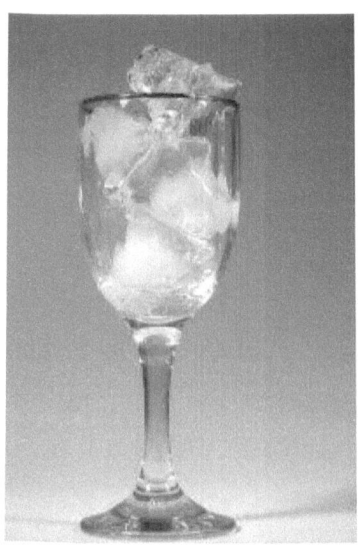

Different Choices

Different rehab centers around the world furnish treatment targeting the whole life of the person at issue rather than simply the symptoms. This demands identifying the base grounds of the dependency and wiping out the same.

Detox centers have healing sessions where the patient is gently guided to open his concerns and fears at the most bass level. This aids in discovering the root cause of the habit.

A positive treatment plan is then worked up enabling the patient to survive his habit and continue towards leading a pleased and sound life.

Alcoholism might result from clinical depression. In these cases treatment has to demand more intensive work on the mind of the person. Psycho therapeutic treatment programs are organized for these people which are an effective alternate treatment for this condition. This treatment works both at the addictive and emotional layer of the patient.

Religious counsel as a treatment option for the condition of alcoholism is as well gaining in fame. Spiritual belief might act as a major motivation for a person to desert his habit of drinking.

Varied meditation techniques instructed by spiritual leaders of several organizations go a long way in assisting addicts defeat stress and attain serenity thereby making it easier for them to desert their habit and start leading a peaceful and calm life.

Techniques include yoga, different types of meditations and trance. Meditation helps a person center inward thereby making the individual ease his mind and turn tension free and unstrained.

When the person is pleased and content with himself, he's not affected by anything happening around him and he no longer requires anything habit-forming to feel pleased, comfortable and peaceful.

Many people are going in for this kind of program as they feel that meditation is better than medication. While medicine is impermanent, meditation supplies one a lasting answer.

Trance work is similarly something like meditation. This helps the person center his brain on studying deeper truths and furnishes the addict with awesome inner strength to help him master his enticements with relative simplicity.

Yoga which is truly popular now is a different effective treatment strategy for the condition of alcoholism. Yoga helps in effectively cutting down stress and tension in a person and relieves him of anxiety. Yoga centers on gentle stretching and yields an effective harmoniousness between the body and the brain.

A different alternative treatment which has been exposed to be effective is called nutritional counseling.

A lot of inadequacies related to nutrition develop due to excessive ingestion of alcohol. The body of the alcoholic stops taking up crucial nutrients which helps the individual in being healthy as his small intestine is no more able to soak up the nutrients necessary.

Nutritional counseling might help after an individual abandons the habit of drinking.

Generally, he or she is assessed for counseling and is apprised of a diet to abide by in order to return to a fit and strong life. This includes the balancing of the sugar level in the blood of the individual who is on the road to recovery.

One more effective alternative treatment includes acupuncture. This has turned out to be successful in numerous cases. Acupuncturists apprise patients to take this as a support treatment along with other treatments.

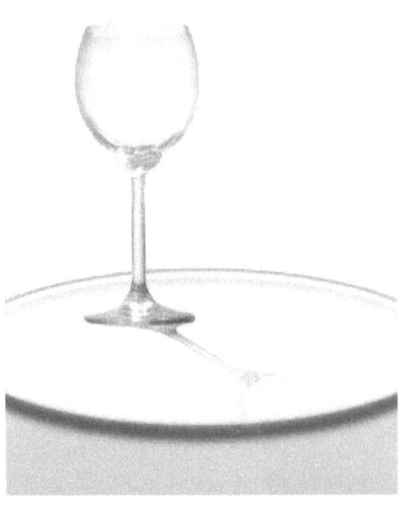

Wrapping Up

This can be a hard journey and there may be time that you slip up... If you do remember this:

- Get right back on track. Quit drinking—the sooner the better.

- Remember, every day is a fresh day to begin over. Although it may be unnerving to slip, you don't have to carry on drinking. You're responsible for your selections.

- Comprehend that setbacks are standard when individuals undertake a huge change. It's your progress in the long haul that counts.

- Don't run yourself down. It does not help. Don't let feelings of disheartenment, angriness, or guilt stop you from asking for help and going back on track.

- Get a little help. Contact your counselor or a sober and supportive acquaintance immediately to talk about what occurred, or go to an AA or other mutual-help meeting.

- Think it over. With a little space, work on your own or with support to better comprehend why the episode occurred at that certain time and place.

- Learn from what came about. Decide what you have to do so that it won't occur again, and write it down. Utilize the experience to beef up your commitment.

- Keep away from triggers to drink. Do away with any alcohol at home. If possible, avoid revisiting the state of affairs in which you drank.

- Discover alternatives. Stay busy with matters that are not affiliated with drinking.

Best of luck in your endeavor.

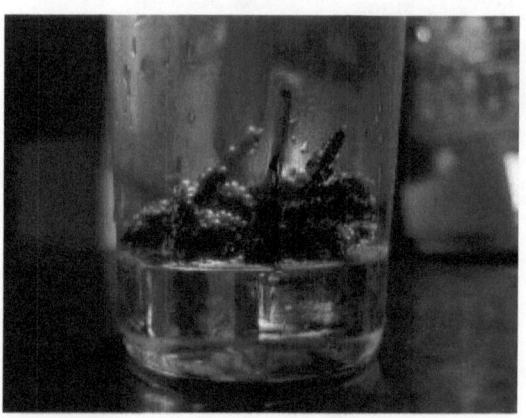